Juicing Bible: Complete Guide to Juicing for Weight Loss

Juicing Detox and Cleanse With Recipes

By: Margo Wilson

PUBLISHERS NOTES

Disclaimer

This publication is intended to provide helpful and informative material. It is not intended to diagnose, treat, cure, or prevent any health problem or condition, nor is intended to replace the advice of a physician. No action should be taken solely on the contents of this book. Always consult your physician or qualified health-care professional on any matters regarding your health and before adopting any suggestions in this book or drawing inferences from it.

The author and publisher specifically disclaim all responsibility for any liability, loss or risk, personal or otherwise, which is incurred as a consequence, directly or indirectly, from the use or application of any contents of this book.

Any and all product names referenced within this book are the trademarks of their respective owners. None of these owners have sponsored, authorized, endorsed, or approved this book.

Always read all information provided by the manufacturers' product labels before using their products. The author and publisher are not responsible for claims made by manufacturers.

Digital Edition

Manufactured in the United States of America

WHAT YOU WILL LEARN IN THIS BOOK

How This Book Will Help You and Why

There is a juicing revolution underway in the world. As more and more persons are starting to find out that juicing is beneficial they are making the transition to include juicing in their diets.

This book is the perfect guide to the world of juicing. All of the benefits are outlined and there are some fantastic juicing recipes for the reader to try. You get to learn which vegetables and fruits are best for juicing and how to shop for juicers.

Dive Right into the Book! Or Learn a Bit More About the Author

Bonus

Thank you for your purchase and to help you on your weight loss journey and becoming healthier, I've arranged for you to get a special report, "*13 Secrets to Accelerated Weight Loss*", to speed you towards your health and fitness goals.

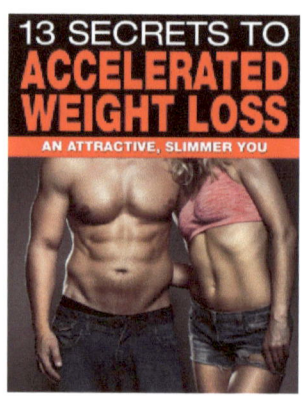

Enter a valid email address and I'll send you your special report as a way of thanking you for buying my book. This report will give you actionable ideas that are simple to use and will help you become a healthier, slimmer version of yourself.

Between the report and what you learn here in this book, you'll have an unbeatable combination to help you reach your goals.

Just go to:

www.getfitwithjuicing.com

Go now and get started!

TABLE OF CONTENTS

DEDICATION

This book is dedicated to my mother. She taught me everything I needed to know about juicing. It is an extremely healthy practice and is a great way to get children the vitamins and nutrients they need.

Chapter 1- Smoothies Or Juices - Which Is Better?

If you are new to the game of juicing, and are lost within your studies of raw fruits and vegetables, then you might be wondering which is better, juices or smoothies. Both can be incredibly delicious, and both can be very healthy, but in the world of being a veggie or fruit vampire, it's very typical for any juicer to want to know every single detail about what he/she is putting into his/her body. So let's do a little comparison, and see what the pros and cons are of both juices and smoothies.

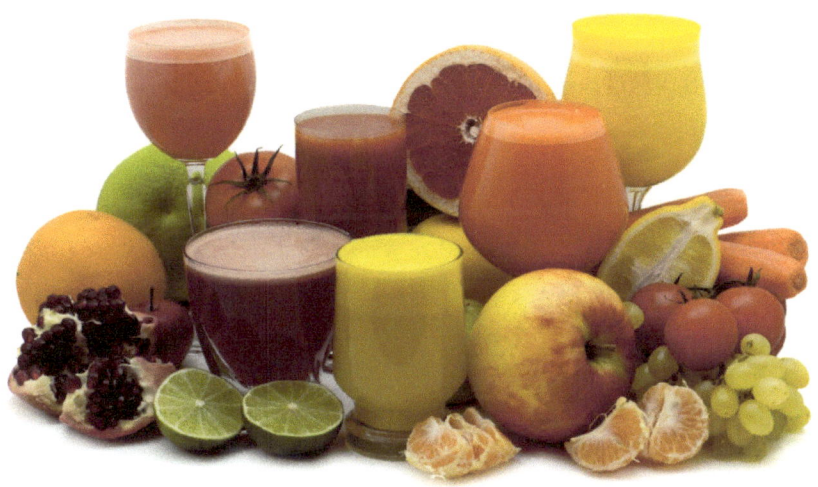

To start with, smoothies are much thicker than your average juice concoction, and sometimes they can be very sweet. Many times they will have added honey for a little bit more of a sugary twist. One might argue that with sugar coated practices like that, smoothies can give anyone a little bit more energy than juices; however, the nutritional value that is extracted from fruits and vegetables in raw form can provide plenty of a boost.

Smoothies also may or may not contain milk, and generally never ice cream. If you are lactose intolerant this could be a problem; except crushed ice can be an easy replacement for any dairy that would otherwise be found in a smoothie. The beauty of a smoothie is that plenty can go into any mix and the taste, if not pleasant, can easily be disguised. With juice this is a little bit harder to do, but there are tricks available to the expert juicer.

Smoothies can be very expensive when purchased pre-made, but someone who chooses to do it him/herself at home can save a pretty penny. This goes for juice making as well. Like your average juices, smoothies can be made from leafy greens if desired, and most smoothie recipes are high in antioxidants, dietary fibre, and vitamins, much like homemade juice.

All in all, there is very little difference between juices and smoothies, and really only in how you prepare them. It comes down to a matter of texture and small pleasure in preference. If you are new to juicing, your best bet would be to try a little of both before settling upon either or, and some people like to switch back and forth. There are plenty of recipe books for both juices and smoothies, and so a great place to start would be there. If something looks appetizing, you really can't know for certain until you try it. Take note of the ingredients and if you are curious, do a little research on the nutritional benefits of each one.

Juicing For Health

Juicing for health is one of the best things that anyone can be doing right now, especially with all of the sicknesses and out of shape bodies that you see and hear about every day. The enzymes, minerals, and vitamins that fruits and vegetables contain can do wonders for a body when the effort to consume them on a daily basis is applied.

All of the benefits that nature's foods contain are designed to fight off certain elements of disease, and each individual fruit and vegetable has its own helpful resources. For instance, celery is known to help with lowering blood pressure and contains eight known anti-cancer compounds. Now imagine all of the hundreds of different types of fruits and vegetables that are out there, and what each one has to offer to the human body. When combined as one - you've got yourself a little magic potion.

Juicing for health purposes is simply just smart. One reason for it being a good idea lies in the fact that a lot of people have poor health of the intestines due to eating poorly. This makes digesting nutrients very inefficient. However, if you condense your fruits and vegetables down to a juice, all of the benefits can be absorbed a lot easier.

Juicing for health is also important, because on average most people don't eat the suggested amount of vegetables. The ideal amount would be about 3 - 5 pounds a day, but most people are unable to consume this amount even in a week. This is partly due to the fact that it is a lot of eating, which can be very time consuming. With a juicer, you can easily take all the work and stress out, and start living a healthier life style immediately.

CHAPTER 2- THE HEALTH BENEFITS OF JUICING

Many people are highly interested in starting a juicing plan, and they are well aware that doing so can be good for the body, but most don't really know what the health benefits of juicing are; well there are tons. In fact so many, that there is no way that they can all be covered in this chapter, but we'll go ahead and take a look at some of the biggest, and most commonly known benefits of juicing.

Leafy greens contain what is known as chemical plant fibre, which is very good for fighting off disease, and is known to thwart major sicknesses. There is also another plus to chemical fibre and that is its ability to help with allergy symptoms in the long term. If ever there were a reason to start juicing, a safe way to combat allergies would be it.

When you eat anything, the liquids from food contain the energy that your body uses. The actual solids are stripped away and become waste, while the liquids are absorbed. Your body is its own juicer. Doesn't seem like a hard concept to grasp until you imagine your body juicing something like a hamburger. There is no reason to be extreme and not enjoy beef every now and then, but one of the benefits of juicing is that it can help with your digestive system, making the absorption easier on your body.

By juicing, it is much easier to get your daily dose of the essential amino acids, which are very necessary for a healthy life style. The amino acids in discussion are basically impossible to receive any other way other than from food, but at the same time, the task of trying to get all of them each and every day can be quite daunting. Juicing makes this much more manageable.

Juicing is a wonderful way to cleanse and restore energy. One of the best benefits of juicing is the fact that if done properly, metabolism, immune system, and energy levels can become well balanced, meaning that you can have the energy you need without feeling as if you are in over drive.

The benefits of juicing are plenty, and yet they are still not completely realized by many people. Have you made the conscience decision to live a better and healthier life? If so, ask yourself why you want to do so and for whom? Is it just for you, or do you wish to keep yourself around for your loved ones as well? Do you want more energy? More time to do things? It may seem so simple a thing, but getting specific with your goals is a great way for anyone to really make progress with his/her actions.

The most common benefit of juicing is the fact that its a great way to get your full serving of fruits and vegetables. Considering that there are many things needed for a healthy diet, and that they are to be consumed on a daily basis, juicing makes it as easy as pie.

Another great plus is the ability to free up time. By doing all of your juicing on the weekends, you can easily store your concoctions in the fridge and reap the rewards throughout the week, while maintaining a healthy, daily life style. Consuming fruits and vegetables takes time, and most people are simply too busy to do so, but drinking them all down, together, is fast and simple.

Finally, probably the biggest benefit of juicing is all of the money that can be saved. For very little you can hit the grocery store, pick out everything you need, and then do your juicing in one go so that you are set up for the rest of the week. Juicing doesn't really require the use of that many fruits and vegetables, especially if you are using an efficient juicer. Unfortunately a lot of people spend tons of money on junk foods that they think will give them energy. Its hard for anyone to imagine that you could get so much energy from a fruit/vegetable drink, but its absolutely true, and you'll have cash to spare.

CHAPTER 3- TIPS FOR BECOMING A HEALTHY JUICER

Knowing your fruits and vegetables very well can help in becoming a healthy juicer. There is a bit of an art to juicing, and though its not rocket science, you have to think of it as cooking, where ratios and flavours are very important. Some absolutely terrible concoctions can be created from bad juicing, and there may be a good chance that you already know this from your own experience. To help you become a smart and healthy juicer, here are some tips you won't want to do without.

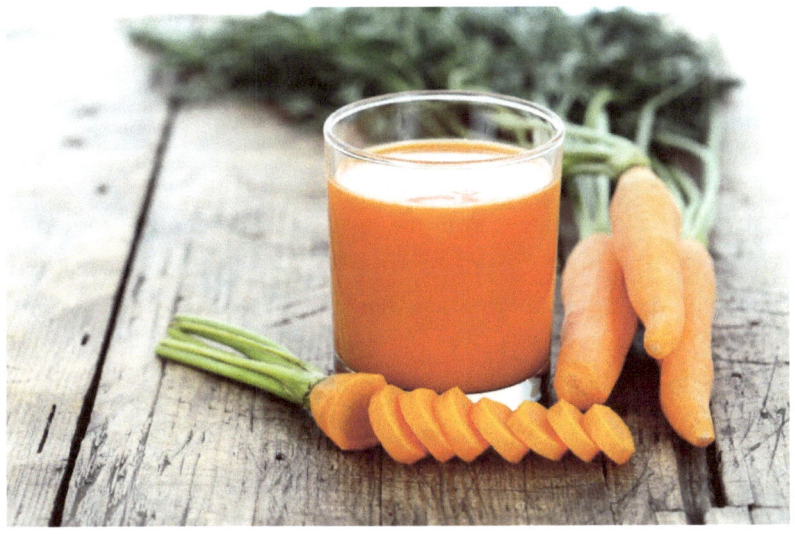

If you are looking for a bite to add to your juices, be careful of ingredients that do this too much. For instance, ginger is used a lot for flavouring and so is lime, but it typically takes very little of either ingredient to add full flavour to a brew. Before you decide to give up on that last terrible juice recipe, you may want to try it again, but lighten up on spices and citruses.

Understand when to peel and when not to peel a fruit. Some people are against eating orange peels because of the dyes that they contain, while others love the spicy zip. Whichever person you are, imagine how much you can throw a juice off by adding certain peels. On the other hand, some peels do not have very much flavouring and can be very good for you.

A little bit of apple is the perfect way to sweeten a drink without having to use sugar.

Depending on the juicer and yourself, juicing can be time consuming every now and then. If you don't want to get into juicing every single day, try juicing 16 ounces instead of the daily 8, and drink two days' worth of juice then. By going about it like this, you can juice about 3 days out of the week, but get a full week's worth of nutrition.

Most people become very eager to get started juicing, and so they go crazy at first. Take it easy if you are new to this, because your digestive system needs time to get used to your new health plan. Consuming too much juice all the time can give you digestive fits.

A lot of recipes will call for carrots and though they are tasty in your drinks, try not to get too carried away with them. Too many carrots all the time can raise a person's blood sugar level quite a bit. A good juicing regime is one that is diverse.

Buy only what you intend to juice, and make sure that it is done within a timely manner. At first it will no doubt take you some time to learn what proportions you will need for your favourite recipes, but once you get the hang of it - try to be a frugal shopper. Too many people stock up on fruits and vegetables, only to find that they can't juice them in a timely manner. The majority of the produce goes bad, and money is blown. Even if this isn't the case, its important to juice everything when its still fresh enough to contain all of the minerals, vitamins, and general nutrition.

Remember that you don't need to wash what you intend to peel. This is something that a lot of juice enthusiasts don't think about, and so this tip can be very helpful for saving time.

CHAPTER 4- JUICE DIET-THE KEY TO PHYSICAL FITNESS

Juicing diets are becoming more and more popular as the thought and desire to get fit and healthy is continually growing in people's heads. With a well-planned and defined juicing diet, anyone can boost their weight loss, or physical fitness efforts, and in the process improve their health. A lot of people think that trying to get your nutrition from raw fruits and vegetables is pardon the pun, "fruitless", but indeed this is completely false.

Vegetables, especially when eaten raw, are much richer in minerals and vitamins, and many of these types of minerals such as iron, and vitamins such as C, can give any one the boost that they need to maintain the energy levels that are required for running, weight lifting, aerobics, cardio, or even something like power walking.

The beauty of a juicing diet is that trying to digest other types of foods can really drag the body down. Juicing diets aren't like this. Raw veggies for instance tend to be a good source of dietary fibre, and are so easy for the digestive system to strip away what isn't needed, that it doesn't leave the body feeling tired. This naturally means that anyone can get going on his/her exercise routine.

A juice diet is naturally better for you, and believe it or not, the different varieties of fruits and vegetables that are available in the world is so diverse, that the combinations and mixtures are virtually endless as well. Its easy for anyone to use this method to figure out what he/she likes by taste, and what his/her body thinks is pleasant as well. Not to mention all of the free radical fighting capabilities of fruits and veggies.

If you decide to do a diet of juice, with the intent of getting an easy health kickback for your getting fit efforts, then you will probably have a smile on your face when you realize all of the healthy things that you are not only doing for your body, but putting into your body as well. Plus, a lot of times someone will start his/her own customized juicing diet and find that doing so helps to regulate his/her body and mood. From bathroom visits, to sleep schedule, one of the best ways to balance the body and mind is to get started on a juicing diet.

Juicing For Weight Loss

Juicing for weight loss is an excellent choice for anyone who wants to get his/her body into better shape. It requires very little effort, is affordable, fast, healthy, and it can be a lot of fun. As mentioned in Chapter 2, fruits and vegetables contain all of the natural vitamins and antioxidants that the human body was meant to consume all along, so it's no surprise that juicing for weight loss is a much more affective substitute to other foods when designing plan.

If you have even the most simple of exercise routines set up, doing a little juicing every day can complement such a routine quite nicely. This is where most people go wrong, and become discouraged. Eating right isn't going to burn away calories on its own. You will need a little bit of activity to go along with your juice, but a little is better than nothing at all.

Juicing for weight loss is a much better substitute than pure fasting. Water Fasting is practically useless, because everyone needs calories and healthy sugars to be turned into energy for movement or exercise. As mentioned before, eating well should not be the only thing that is part of a health plan.

Another great benefit of juicing for weight loss is the fact that everything you will be putting into your body is highly concentrated and pure. There are no dietary fats with juicing, and you will get all of the minerals, enzymes, and vitamins that your body truly needs to maintain a balanced metabolism. Not to mention the enormous boost that your immune system gets, which of course is extremely helpful when trying to fight off the common cold.

If you are just getting started with your goal for a healthier life, and are seriously considering making juicing a part of your daily schedule, here's a great tip. Before you start your exercising, take a week or so to do a juice fast. This will clean out your system, while storing precious energy to get you going and make you feel like a million bucks when you do start exercising.

CHAPTER 5- A WIDE VARIETY OF VEGETABLES, FRUITS & HERBS FROM WHICH TO CHOOSE

Cabbage

Its good in coleslaw, in stir fry, and the sometimes multi-coloured leafy green that can be found worldwide known as cabbage has some major health perks.

Cabbage contains an excellent source of Glutamine, which is a non-essential amino acid that is necessary during illness or even injury, as it can be found in circulation through the blood stream. Cabbage also contains large amounts of vitamin C, an antioxidant that works beautifully to produce collagens, boost the immune system, and help scrapes and gashes heal faster.

Cabbage is also known to help with things like stomach ulcers, arthritis, aging, and it is chock full of Iodine, which helps to balance and maintain the central nervous symptom. On a side note, cabbage is believed to help with the effects of Alzheimer's disease.

Cabbage also contains good amounts of vitamin B6, which works in the conversion process of Tryptophan and Serotonin, which might help in the balance of sleep and mood.

Wheatgrass

Wheatgrass juice contains extremely high quantities of chlorophyll, and is jam packed with essential minerals. It is lovingly referred to as one of the super foods, and is harvested before it reaches its full maturity as ordinary wheatgrass. This occurs when the wheatgrass first begins jointing, and it is at this stage that it is at its nutritional prime.

Wheatgrass juicing is a perfect for anyone who is looking for a kick of energy to make his/her body and mind feel balanced. You have the high amounts of chlorophyll to thank for this, which is the same nutrient in plants that is developed by the sun's energy.

Wheatgrass juice provides a good source of many minerals such as calcium, protein, and iron, but it also contains good amounts of magnesium, which is a necessary element for a calm mind, and more positive attitude.

It is also thought to be helpful with Alzheimer's disease, the immune system, and extremely beneficial to the blood stream. No matter its uses, it cannot be disputed that wheatgrass is a healthy thing to take into the human body, but beware of all of the claims of what it can do, because many are unproven.

However, if you are looking for a great source of amino acids, minerals, enzymes, and vitamins (C, E, and B12), then you may want to further explore the quickly growing and interesting world of wheatgrass juicing.

Tomato

The tomato is a member of the nightshade family, whose origins go back to South America. Often mistaken as a vegetable, a tomato is actually a fruit, because of the fact that the seeds during the growing process are contained within the final result, stemming from the ovary of the flower itself.

Tomatoes come in all shapes, sizes, and colours and are enjoyed throughout the world. They also have many health benefits, partly due to their contents of antioxidants. Tomatoes have what is called lycopene, which is believed to at times help with prostate cancer. Tomatoes also have been known to contain large amounts of both vitamin A as well as vitamin C. Studies have even shown that tomatoes may help with heart disease and blood pressure.

Because the tomato contains decent levels of a healthy sugar, this can also be a better alternative than regular sugar, and tomatoes also contain small amounts of carbohydrates, which makes adding them to a pasta dish very delightful without packing on added carbs.

Carrot

Carrots are a great vegetable in the sense that the ways in which you can use them is quite diverse. From gourmet feasts fit for a king, to a simple peanut butter combo snack, there is no denying the enjoyable snack of a carrot, but they also can be quite good for the human body.

The famous orange colour of most carrots is caused by the presence of beta-carotene, which is later transferred to vitamin A in the intestines. Vitamin A makes up the majority of the nutritional value of carrots, which is good for vision, bone health, skin health and the immune system.

Other minerals and vitamins that are taken in by the body when consuming carrots are: iron, magnesium, B6, Vitamin C, and Calcium; but there are many more that are also good for the body. A lack of vitamin A can actually lead to blindness, but at the same time eating too many carrots can cause the skin to take on an orange colour.

For many juicers and many juicing recipes, carrots are a huge ingredient, generally acting as a staple for many juice concoctions. The flavour of carrots works quite well when combined with a spice like ginger, and the combination of carrots to apples to ginger is a nutritious and absolutely delicious drink.

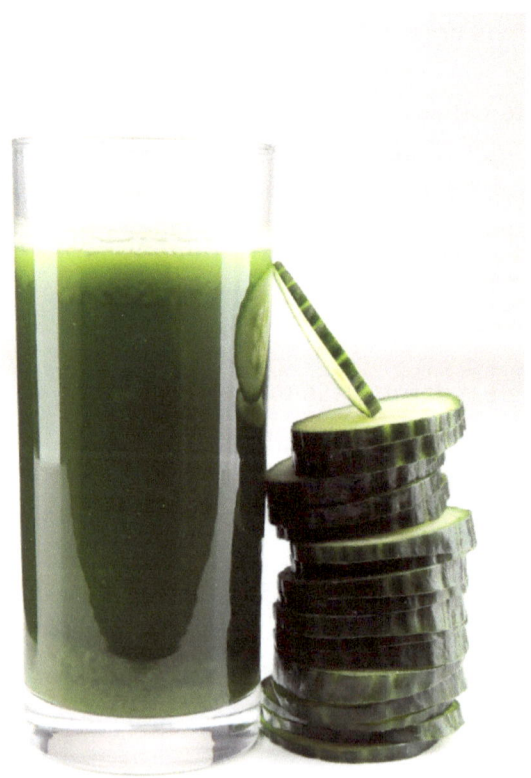

English Cucumber

English cucumbers, or Burpless cucumbers, throw a lot of people off because most have never even heard of one before. So what's the lowdown on this interestingly named veggie? First, you may be surprised to know that there are about one hundred different kinds of cucumbers (cucumis sativus for those who want the Latin name), and that most cucumbers have different purposes. Certain varieties are used mainly for pickles, while others work much better if they are fresh and used in things like salads.

The differences between the English cucumber and the one that most people know of aren't that prominent for the most part. English cucumbers tend to have less seeds, and are much easier on the digestive system and because of their packaging - they tend to be easier to cut and require no peeling, so you can throw them into whatever, right off the bat.

Because they are easier to digest, they are often times referred to as Burpless cucumbers, and as gross as the name is - its quite true. Also, for those who detect a slightly bitter taste in cucumbers, because the English cucumber has less seeds, the bitter taste should be greatly reduced.

In terms of health benefits, this vegetable certainly has its fair share, containing high amounts of vitamin C, vitamin B6, potassium, pantothenic acid or B5, and Magnesium, just to name a few. People who are having urinary problems may find that cucumbers help, as they promote the flow of urine. They are also good for liver problems, pancreatic issues, and can help the body digest protein a little better, so if you are going the vegan route, you may want to make any cucumber a part of your daily eating routine.

Considering that the English cucumber like many other varieties contains mostly water, eating these veggies can be a great way to properly hydrate the body. Silica can also be found, which is good for strengthening connective tissues. Any kind of cucumber is good for skin care, and considering that they are so low in calories, and yet have good fibre content - a great vegetable to add to any diet plan would easily be the English cucumber.

Celery

Celery is one of those things that are hard to do without in a daily diet, especially if you are trying to lose weight, you might want to consider making celery apart of your eating schedule. Celery contains a very fibrous, low calorie content, which can aid in filling a person up, without all of the digestive side effects. If you are a vegan or vegetarian, you still need calcium. Celery is ideal for people who don't want to eat meat or would rather avoid dairy products because it supplies a good source of calcium.

Celery also contains a light form of salt, which can be easily digested by people who are sensitive to salts. Celery juice itself is also believed to sometimes help with pain, or more specifically arthritis in the joints.

As a last note, it's very important to be aware that celery has been labelled as a major allergen, and depending upon the person, the reaction could be quite severe. If you have tried celery before and have had no problem with it, then you already know that you will be fine, but if you haven't - you may want to be cautious.

Orange

There are many different types of oranges and varieties in the world, but no matter the one you have, one thing's for certain - oranges are an incredible source of vitamins and minerals. In fact, the orange is widely accepted as one of the most beneficial fruits available to the human diet, and eating this fruit on a daily basis could very well help to combat some possibly serious health issues.

Vitamin C makes up the majority of the nutritious value of the citrus fruit, which is lacking in most people's diet, though this very strong antioxidant is a must, and some creatures such as bats cannot live without it.

The orange like most things healthy contains very few calories, but it has a good dose of carbs for energy, and as most fruits do - contains good forms of sugars for a boost. Orange juice in the morning has been known to give an edge to awareness and focus, and if its made a staple at breakfast time, then a person can be ready for just about anything.

Some of the other vitamins and minerals that the orange sports in its genetic makeup are calcium, zinc, magnesium, B6, phosphorus, potassium, foliate, niacin, and thiamine.

The health benefits of oranges are pretty diverse as this citrus fruit has been known to aid in problems with digestion, cholesterol, kidney stones, heart disease, and naturally the immune system. If the old saying "an apple a day keeps the doctor away" is true, then perhaps we should also learn to include in that phrase the orange.

Apple

The apple is a fruit belonging to the rose family that has made appearances across time, ranging from ancient Greek mythology to the bible itself. It would almost seem that the apple is the oldest thing on earth, but unlike the poisoned version in Snow White, the fruit that we are aware of is far healthier for you.

Ironically in comparison to other fruits, apples actually have a very low amount of vitamin C, but health benefits are still much greater than many other types of fruits. If you have irritable bowels, or find yourself constipated, apples are great for the digestive track, plus if you are trying to lose weight and need something to snack on other than candy, apples are very good for cholesterol and helping with weight loss.

By adding a little peanut butter to the fruit, you can have a healthy source of protein and all the minerals and antioxidants that your body needs. Vitamin B6, calcium, zinc, iron, potassium, magnesium, and foliate is just some of the things that the apple has to offer.

Apples are also widely believed to help with mental issues or instability, and apparently can aid in cognitive processes which may be helpful to elderly persons and preventing "mental aging". Apples also are thought to be good for the bone density in post-menopausal women, helping in strengthening the bones against osteoporosis.

Apples also have the ability to lower the body's need for insulin, which in turn could be of great use to diabetics.

Beet

The beet has a long history of cultivation, going way back some 2 millennium BC. Some people like, and some people absolutely despise the taste, but like them or not - they are very healthy to eat.

Long ago beets were used to help problems with constipation, but beets are now being recognized as being able to reduce blood pressure very quickly. The ancient Romans used beets to calm fevers, and as they are full of carbohydrates, but low in calories - they are an awesome supply of healthy energy.

Like many other fruits and vegetables, beets are packed full of good vitamins and minerals such as iron, vitamin A, C, potassium, magnesium and calcium. Beat juice is also good for liver health, including diabetic liver, and have been known to lower cholesterol levels in some individuals.

The taste of beets can be very overpowering for some when juicing, but this flavour can usually be tamed by adding a simple ingredient such as carrots, assuming that the ratios are right.

Garlic

They've been known to keep vampires at bay, as well as other people, but did you know that garlic not only brings a lot of zest to pasta dishes but is also quite healthy?

Garlic has played an important role in folklore medicine for centuries, and its uses were quite broad. It is been known to be used as a repellent for pesky mosquitos, which may be where the whole idea of keeping vampires away comes from.

Garlic in general can be a very powerful antibiotic, but beware because some people can also be quite allergic to it. However if you can manage to take it even in supplemental form, you will find that it can be very beneficial to the body.

Garlic contains large amounts of vitamin C and B6, as well as minerals like calcium, zinc, potassium, iron, panothenic acid, magnesium and phosphorus

Ginger

Ginger is one of the most famous and beloved spices, especially by avid juicers, because ginger can bring a lot of flavour to most anything, but did you know that ginger is very good for you?

It was used in folk medicine for years all over the world, and has many benefits. Sometimes Ginger has been used to combat some forms of diarrhoea, morning sickness, and heartburn.

Ginger has a lot to offer when it comes to helping with headaches, motion sickness, and is thought to be an excellent flu preventive. Ginger is very soothing for stomach related issues and in some ancient cultures it was used for menstrual cramping.

Ginger also works well to thin the blood and keep the blood stream healthy, which can help with the overall health of the heart. In some scenarios it is believed to have helped with fevers, and adding a little ginger to honey and lemon in hot water, makes for an excellent and long term healthy tea.

CHAPTER 6- 11 SIMPLE JUICING RECIPES

If you just bought a juicer for the first time and you need some quick juicing recipes to get started, without becoming overwhelmed - look no further. Here are eleven easy, tasty, and healthy juicing recipes that no first time juicer should do without.

Basic Carrot Juice

Simply juice 5 to 6 carrots and enjoy. Carrots provide a wonderful source of strength for bones, teeth, hair, skin, and are also very cleansing for the liver.

Pepper Juice

Ingredients:

- 1 red pepper
- ½ cucumber
- 4 celery stalks
- 1 green pepper
- Pinch of black pepper

Apple Milk Shake (without the milk)

Ingredients:

- 1 banana
- 1 tablespoon brewer's yeast
- ½ of a peeled orange
- 1 - 2 apples

The Body Boost

Ingredients:

- 3 carrots
- 2 apples
- 1 part ginger

Delicious and revitalizing!

The Mouth Waterer

Ingredients:

- 4 parts apple
- 1 parts watermelon
- 2 parts pineapple

Make sure to remove any seeds first.

Simple Beat Hybrid

Ingredients:

- 1 beet
- 1 stalk of celery
- 1 carrot
- 1 small part of ginger
- 1 apple

Stomach Settling Juice

Ingredients:

- 2 kiwis
- ½ head of cabbage
- 1 beet

Tomato Vampire

Ingredients:

- 2 tomatoes
- 2 sprigs of parsley
- 2 apples
- 1 garlic clove

Orange Delight

Ingredients:

- 2 oranges
- 2 carrots
- ½ cup of dandelion heads
- ½ lemon

Ginger Ale

Ingredients:

- Sparkling mineral water
- 1 sliced apple
- ½ cup of grapes
- ½ inch of fresh ginger

- ¼ lemon
- ½ lime

Cherry Berry Madness

Ingredients:

- ¾ cup of blueberries
- ½ cup of pitted cherries
- 1 apple

Chapter 7- Factors To Consider When Buying A Juicer

Getting into juicing is a really exceptional way to maintain your health, increase your immune system, and simply put, live a healthier life style. When most people make the decision to start juicing, they assume that all juicers are the same, when in reality, they aren't.

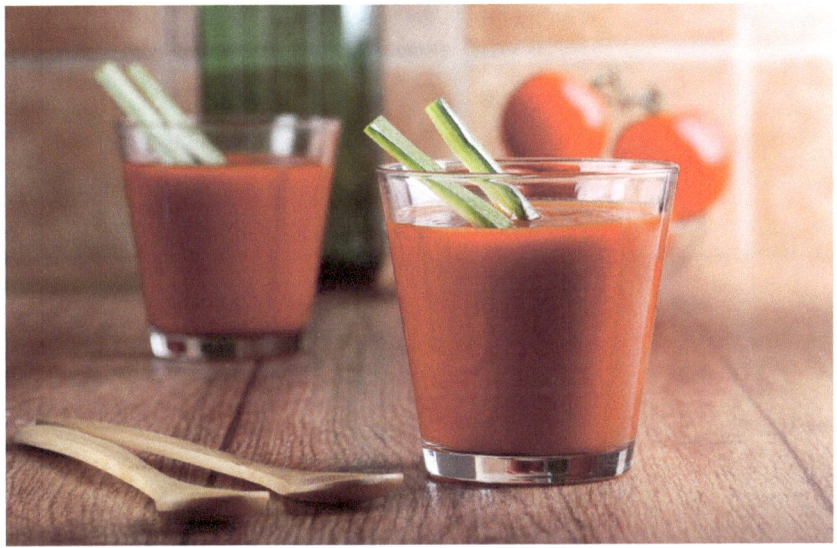

Buying a juicer should be a simple task, and as long as you are armed with the right knowledge it can be. However, it is pointless to shill out any money for a juicer that won't meet your needs. For the best experience as a first time juicer buyer, please read this chapter thoroughly.

Price

Juicers vary in price, and no matter what your budget is, just because you may be able to afford an expensive juicer, doesn't necessarily mean that it's the best one.

In fact, there are a good number of much cheaper models that are way more efficient in doing their job. In all honesty, you can get a very good juicer for less than $500, with a lot of variation of price within that amount.

Size

Some juicers are monstrous in size, while others aren't very big at all. Consider the fact that one with all the bells and whistles will no doubt have to be larger to accommodate such features.

Take into consideration your counter space, or where ever you plan to rest your juicer. Make sure to read the dimensions on the box of each one that you consider buying.

Maintenance

For you it may be best to find a juicer that is very easy to maintain. The maintenance will pretty much be just cleaning by washing and drying, but a juicer that has a lot of parts, or hard to reach parts is obviously going to be more of a chore to take care of.

A good juicer with a respected reputation will make known to the consumer all that is involved in the cleaning and preparation.

Purpose

Define how you plan to use your juicer, and therefor what you want it to do for you. A great place to start is with a health or fitness plan if you are headed in that direction.

Will you be juicing mostly vegetables, fruits, or wheatgrass? Wheatgrass juicers are very specific for what they do, and not all juicers can juice both vegetables and fruits, so make sure that you know the true potential of the model that you are interested in; I will discuss this matter in greater detail in the upcoming chapter.

CHAPTER 8- SPECIALIZED JUICERS- WHAT TYPE SHOULD YOU BUY?

Should You Get A Manual Juicer?

If you're in the market for a manual juicer, there is a good chance that you have some questions that need answering. There are a lot of different types of juicers to do research on, and there are certainly many, many different kinds of manual juicers.

Manual juicers can vary in their effectiveness when squeezing fruits. In order to maintain the easiest possible use, a juicer like this must be built in such a manner that a lot of force can be brought down upon the fruit. Think about it. Should you be trying to apply 1 - 2 thousand pounds of pressure, or should the juicer? In order for the manual juicer to do this, it requires the right kind of construction and materials, which means that they can sometimes weigh too much for practical kitchen use.

If you plan to squeeze nothing but limes, oranges, and lemons, then this kind of a juicer may be ideal for you, but if you are looking for something that can give you the choice of saying "I think I'm going to try juicing this now", then you should probably go with an electric juicer that can handle many different types of fruits, as well as veggies.

If you're ok with that thought, and all you want is to juice oranges per say, then make sure that you read accurate reviews from others who have purchased manual juicers to ensure that you find one that produces a good yield of juice, doesn't require a lot of effort, is easy to clean (they usually are), and is easy enough to operate to the point where it doesn't take you 2 hours to juice a couple of oranges.

Should You Get A fruit Juicer?

Fruit juicers are an awesome way to get your vitamins, or to simply get started with juicing in general. If you are a bit of a "fruit" about fruit, then there should really be nothing holding you back from making juice for better life style, and consumption habits. Still, if you are reading this and you haven't actually bought a fruit juicer yet, then perhaps you should take into account just a few things before handing over the cash.

Decide upon what you think you will be juicing the most, as obviously if you are interested in raw vegetables - this kind of juicer isn't going to cut it for you.

What's your budget? If you spend too low on anything, you may get something that is junky and practically useless or breaks right off the bat. If you think that you would find something in a slightly higher dollar price range, you might be better off getting a multi-purpose juicer instead.

Make sure that when you are looking at fruit juicers that you find out what the clean-up is like. How long should it take you, what's involved, and can any parts be put into a dish washer? These are all legitimate questions to ask yourself.

Not every fruit is the same, so make sure that the juicer that has caught your hungry eye isn't going to disappoint, and will be powerful enough to handle tougher fruits.

How long is the warranty? This is always a must just in case something happens, and in fact, when shopping for any juicer period, you should always pay attention to the warranty and what it covers. A fruit juicer that is on the up and up should have a decent warranty that will cover the essentials in case something happens.

Should You Get A Juicer Mixer Grinder?

Juicer mixer grinders are sometimes thought of as the ultimate multi-function kitchen appliance, having the ability to act as a juicer, mixer, and grinder in an all-in-one structured machine. The concept is wonderful, but is the functionality, or to be more specific - how would such an appliance function with your life style? Before jumping right in and buying one, consider the facts, then assess why you would need this type of mixer, and how you would use it.

The grinder function of a basic juicer mixer grinder combo is typically best suited for grinding coffee beans, nuts, and sometimes for helping with the production of pastas, while the other obvious features are more straight forward and obvious.

The juicer should be powerful enough to juice a large variety of fruits and vegetables, but you also must remember that here is a machine that is designed for several uses, which in turn can cause the machine to falter in one of those uses in specific.

When it comes to the juicer part of the juicer mixer grinder, its pointless to end up with something that is going to produce overtly frothing juices with little yield, leaving you with wastefully moist pulp, and a lot of clean up.

Your best bet may be to truly define what you need the most, and then buy something specific like a grinder for grinding, juicer for juicing, mixer for mixing etc. The luxury of having them all in one package is a nice idea, but it may be harder to find something like this that actually works.

If you shop around, you can no doubt find juicers, mixers, and grinders that are well-built, produce results, are small enough for your kitchen, and won't cost you an arm and a leg.

Should You Buy A Manual Wheatgrass Juicer

Buying a manual wheatgrass juicer can be a tough decision to make, because for one there are so many to take into consideration and two, is it really worth the money? A wheatgrass juicer can be an excellent and well used investment for the kitchen, but before making that big decision and wasting your money, you should probably ask yourself some questions first.

First of all the one great thing about this kind of a juicer is that they obviously don't use up any electricity, so that of course is an instant plus. Also because of this you can be guaranteed that a manual wheatgrass juicer won't make any noise, or at least so much noise that you can't live with it.

You shouldn't however purchase one if you want to be able to juice a wide variety of fruits and vegetables. Wheatgrass juicers are capable of really only handling soft greens and small fruits. If you need something that can do it all, you may want to see the Breville BJE200XL.

Though the daily recommended intake for wheatgrass juice is small, the taste is not exactly enjoyed by all who try it. If you have yet to taste it, please sample some from a friend or family member who has a wheatgrass juicer, before committing to buy one. If you find out that you don't like it, it's not the end of the world, as other types of juicing practices can yield a lot of nutritional benefits.

You may even consider finding a multi-purpose juicer that can handle wheatgrass as well. This particular machine is of course electrical, but if you do the research it is very easy to find one that is powerful, yet not obtrusively noisy.

Since a wheatgrass juicer is such a specific thing to purchase as it only has one true purpose, your best bet really may be in going with a multi-purpose juicer instead.

Should You Buy An Orange Juicer?

Its delicious, its healthy, and first thing in the morning it certainly can give you that pep that you need to tackle life throughout the day. What is it? Its orange juice!

Orange juice is loaded with an extremely high amount of vitamin C, which helps to boost the immune system, and fight things like the flu and the common cold. It doesn't end there because orange juice is also considered to help with lowering cholesterol, boosting blood circulation, and can be a natural aid and substitute to other beverages (soda, alcohol) for weight loss.

At this point you may be salivating at the thought of sinking your pearly whites into an unpeeled orange right now. You may even be thinking that you will bypass this crazy idea, head down to the grocery store, stock up on some cartons of orange juice, and load yourself up on a little vitamin C. Well what if I told you that you could be a little more creative than that, and make your own orange juice right in your very own kitchen?

You can order an orange juicer for practically nothing and mainly because they are simple in design, easy to use, have very few parts, and are designed for simply extracting all the nutrients that your body craves. On average these bad guys will run you around thirty bucks, but beware! You may want to abandon the plastic models and go with something a little bit sturdier.

If you're feeling really enthusiastic, you may want to go with something like a centrifugal electric juicer, which can handle all sorts of raw fruits and vegetables. Usually these things are high powered, and are fast, meaning you can make juice faster than you can drink it. All you'll have to do is peel each orange, cut the inside down into smaller pieces and feed it in.

CHAPTER 9- TOP 3 BEST JUICER PICKS

The best juicer for anyone is one that can perform, does what you need, is easy to maintain, and doesn't take a life time to clean up every time you want to use it. Below is a list of our top 3 best juicer picks, based on price, clean-up, effectiveness, size, and overall performance.

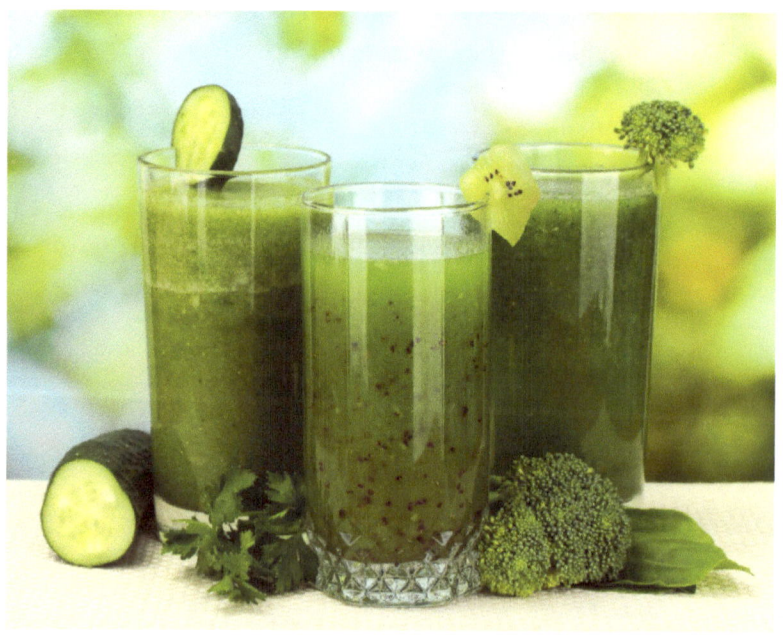

The Breville BJE200XL Compact Juice Fountain

The Breville BJE200XL is by far the more superior of the juicers that I have seen. With 700 watts of power operating at 14,000 RPM, you can enjoy an 8 ounce glass of juice in just five seconds, which puts most juicers to shame.

It has a sleek look, isn't too large or heavy, and the motor is quiet enough to not disturb your home environment, even with all of that wattage. There's practically nothing the BJE200XL Juice Fountain Compact can't do, from handling leafy greens to pulverizing pineapple, with the rind on!

Clean-up of the Breville Compact juicer is also painless, as it can be done quickly and efficiently (less than a couple of minutes) and all of the parts on this Breville Juicer are dishwasher safe, so you need not worry about that.

The centralized pulp container can handle juicing up to 1.5 quarts before needing to be emptied. Very nice for those of us who don't want to clean it out every time we juice something. The Breville BJE200XL Compact Juice Fountain also features a really great, 3 inch feeding tube. This allows the owner to feed in whole fruits and vegetables.

Everyone I've spoken with who uses the Breville BJE200XL also speaks highly of it, and most of these people are experienced juicers - putting the Breville high above any other juicer on their list. This could be partly due to the fact that the BJE200XL - Juice Fountain Compact is designed in such a way that the parts need little maintenance, as they are more resistant to gunk left behind from fruits and vegetables. It comes with a custom brush for easy clean-up, and overall, this thing is built for durability.

When its all said and done you might think that it would cost you an arm and a leg, but it is in fact way cheaper than most other juicers. Though prices can vary, you should expect to pay no more than $130.00.

The Hamilton Beach 67650H Big Mouth Pro Juice Extractor

The Hamilton Beach 67650H Big Mouth Pro Juice Extractor is a one of a kind juicer that is both efficient, and affordable. With a 1.1 horsepower motor, 3 inch wide feeding tube, and a juice cup capable of containing up to 20 ounces of juice, the Hamilton Beach 67650H certainly gives most juicers in its bracket a run for their money.

This one is almost a no brainer, considering that it is one of the nicest and cheapest juicers on the market that can still out perform even some of the more expensive models. One of the bigger perks about it is its small dimensions and weight. Its easy to handle, a breeze to clean up, and simple to put away if need be.

Like all other respectable juicers it comes with a customized cleaning brush to make wash up a piece of cake. All the removable parts on the Hamilton Beach 67650H Big Mouth Pro Juice Extractor are dishwasher safe, and in return make the work load not so bad for clean-up time.

As with any well-built, inexpensive juicer, the 67650H does have a few drawbacks. Softer fruits and vegetables tend to cause more leftover waste. The pulp when juicing certain fruits and veggies can often times be left extremely moist, which means that at times the 67650H produces a slightly unsatisfactory yield in juice.

The other small problem lies in the 1.1 horsepower motor. As you can imagine, this juicer isn't exactly quiet, although it shouldn't be so bad that it wakes the neighbours up.

If you are trying to cut corners and stick to a budget, but don't want to have to sacrifice speed, power, and quality - you may want to consider picking up the Hamilton Beach 67650H Big Mouth Pro Juice Extractor.

The Omega J8005 Juicer

The Omega J8005 Single Gear Commercial Masticating Juicer is for anyone who wants a juicer that can do many jobs. With its small size and versatility, the J8005 is perfect for any kitchen.

It sports a low 80 RPM, 1/3 horsepower motor that can mince just about anything you throw at it. The benefit of having it operate at 80 RPMs is that it won't clog, it won't foam, and there will be no heat build-up, meaning that you will still be able to receive the full nutrition that your fruits and vegetables originally had.

The yield of juice from the Omega J8005 Multi-Purpose Juicer/Food Process Chrome is much greater than most other juicers, and the ability to be able to use if for wheatgrass juicing is another major plus in this machine.

With the Omega J8005 you can also turn out your own pastas with the pasta nozzles, grind coffee beans, flour, make your own baby food, and much more. Despite its ability to be able to do all of these different things, you might assume that the Omega J8005 would be a challenge to clean, but actually this is the complete opposite. Tests show that cleaning and maintenance of this juicer is a piece of cake.

It is also extremely quiet compared to other juicers, making your home environment just as pleasant as it was before. It also sports a nifty feature that is a little harder to find in most commercial juicers. It actually has an auto eject feature for pulp, so you don't have to keep stopping and starting. If you have any problems with the Omega J8005 it comes backed with a 10 year warranty which is also a nice touch.

The price of the Omega J8005 is also very good for what you get, making it one of the better juicers in the below $400 bracket.

If you are looking for a multi-function powerful juicer that can be used for other things on down the road - the Omega J8005 Multi-Purpose Juicer/Food Process Chrome may be perfect for you.

ABOUT THE AUTHOR

Margo Wilson grew up on healthy juices that her mother used to prepare for her. She was a picky eater so her mother ensured that the juices she gave to her had all the nutrients that she would need to get her through the day. She also found that juicing was beneficial to not only help keep her body working properly but it also prevented her from gaining excess weight.

Margo introduced others who were not keen on eating salads and fruits to juicing. They would get what they needed without having to chew and swallow a plate of fruits and veggies. It was so successful that she went ahead to write a book on the benefits of juicing.